Essential Oils
30 Homemade Natural Toothpaste Recipes

Table of content

Introduction

There you stand in another toothpaste aisle, driven there by the sheer fact you are out of toothpaste. You know you don't think much about toothpaste, or the benefits that you are supposed to be getting from your toothpaste. You know you need something that is going to clean, but what about all of those other things they say you ought to have in your toothpaste?

They say that you need to whiten your teeth, but how white your teeth are does nothing for the health of your teeth, so you need to make sure you have something that is going to get rid of the germs, bacteria, and other bad things you don't want in your mouth.

You need something that is going to keep cavities at bay, and hopefully help in the healing of any cavity that you already have. They say that you can't heal any of the cavities that you already have, but this is not actually true. You can heal yourself, maybe not entirely, but who's to say that it can't happen?

The more you take care of yourself, the more your body is going to respond, so you are going to get the results that you want through persistence. There is no gain to giving up, and when you let yourself go, you are going to run into the problems that come with it.

The essential oil toothpastes are going to help you in so many ways, you are going to be amazed that a toothpaste can do so much for you. Sure, the main benefit is going to come with your teeth, but we absorb things with our gums, so even if you don't swallow, you are going to get all kinds of benefits that you never before knew you could.

This book is going to show you how to make all kinds of toothpastes that are not only good for you, but are excellent for your teeth. You are going to get so many different benefits from these oils, whether it come from whiter teeth, better breath, or just a healthier mouth all together. You are going to see the benefits with your gums, your teeth, and even in your mood.

So what are you waiting for? You know you put off that trip to the dentist more than you should.

Now you can go in there and smile with confidence.

Chapter 1 – The Best of the Basics

When it comes to making your own toothpaste, there are a few things you need to keep in mind. The first of which is the fact that you are going to use the same base for all of your pastes. This is because this is the best base you can use for your brushing, as it is going to clean your teeth, help whiten, and stave off those cavities that like to creep on in.

So, in the recipes to follow, you are going to see that in each recipe you need to include the 'toothpaste base' which is the recipe I am going to include right here.

Mix all of these ingredients well in your blender before you add in the oils, and you will end up with an incredible toothpaste, every time.

Toothpaste Base

What you will need:

1 cup baking soda

Coconut oil (add a little at a time until the texture is that of toothpaste)

1 teaspoons Himalayan sea salt (I know the taste can be a bit strong, so feel free to cut it back a bit, just make sure you add some because the health benefits that come with this salt are incredible)

Filtered water (this is to cut down on the oil that you use, though you may prefer to use more oil than water so I'll leave it up to you.)

Directions:

Combine all of the ingredients in a blender and blend until smooth. Now, you are going to start with the baking soda and the salt in the blender first, then add 3 tablespoons of the coconut oil. Watch to get the consistency that you want, and if you want to change and add water instead of more oil, you can do that as well.

When you are using water, make sure you use filtered or purified, without any additives. You don't want to use tap water as there are a lot of extra things added to this water that you don't want to put on your teeth.

As I already said, blend until you are happy with the consistency.

Make sure there are no lumps!

Best Basic Toothpaste

What you will need:

10 drops peppermint oil

5 drops thieves oil

5 drops lemon oil

Toothpaste base

Directions:

Combine all of the ingredients in a bowl, mixing well. Make sure your toothpaste base has been thoroughly mixed before you add in the oils, as there are times when the base remains lumpy, and that is difficult to use to brush with. Once combined, transfer into a small, watertight jar until you are ready to use!

To use, simply dip your toothbrush in the paste and brush as you normally would, then rinse and spit when you are done.

The Tooth Fairy's Delight

What you will need:

10 drops spearmint oil

10 drops rose oil

5 drops lemon oil

Toothpaste base

Directions:

Combine all of the ingredients in a bowl, mixing well. Make sure your toothpaste base has been thoroughly mixed before you add in the oils, as there are times when the base remains lumpy, and that is difficult to use to brush with. Once combined, transfer into a small, watertight jar until you are ready to use!

To use, simply dip your toothbrush in the paste and brush as you normally would, then rinse and spit when you are done.

The Dentist's Choice

What you will need:

10 drops peppermint oil

5 drops clove oil

5 drops ginger oil

Toothpaste base

Directions:

Combine all of the ingredients in a bowl, mixing well. Make sure your toothpaste base has been thoroughly mixed before you add in the oils, as there are times when the base remains lumpy, and that is difficult to use to brush with. Once combined, transfer into a small, watertight jar until you are ready to use!

To use, simply dip your toothbrush in the paste and brush as you normally would, then rinse and spit when you are done.

The Clean Machine

What you will need:

5 drops lemon oil

10 drops peppermint oil

5 drops tea tree oil

5 drops clove oil

Toothpaste base

Directions:

Combine all of the ingredients in a bowl, mixing well. Make sure your toothpaste base has been thoroughly mixed before you add in the oils, as there are times when the base remains lumpy, and that is difficult to use to brush with. Once combined, transfer into a small, watertight jar until you are ready to use!

To use, simply dip your toothbrush in the paste and brush as you normally would, then rinse and spit when you are done.

The Cavinator

What you will need:

10 drops mint oil

5 drops lemon oil

5 drops garlic oil

Toothpaste base

Directions:

Combine all of the ingredients in a bowl, mixing well. Make sure your toothpaste base has been thoroughly mixed before you add in the oils, as there are times when the base remains lumpy, and that is difficult to use to brush with. Once combined, transfer into a small, watertight jar until you are ready to use!

To use, simply dip your toothbrush in the paste and brush as you normally would, then rinse and spit when you are done.

The Pearl Power Paste

What you will need:

10 drops clove oil

10 drops peppermint oil

5 drops myrrh oil

Toothpaste base

Directions:

Combine all of the ingredients in a bowl, mixing well. Make sure your toothpaste base has been thoroughly mixed before you add in the oils, as there are times when the base remains lumpy, and that is difficult to use to brush with. Once combined, transfer into a small, watertight jar until you are ready to use!

To use, simply dip your toothbrush in the paste and brush as you normally would, then rinse and spit when you are done.

Chapter 2 – The Best Whitening Pastes

With the pressure on to have the best teeth around, you aren't going to want to skimp out on any of these pastes. Not only do they taste great, but they are excellent choices when it comes to your teeth health and your gums.

You are going to love the whitening that takes place with any one of these options, not to mention the fact that they taste great and add healthy gum benefits as well.

Do keep in mind with these blends that there is an added ingredient... hydrogen peroxide. Hydrogen peroxide is an excellent teeth whitener, and it is the perfect addition to any home made paste you want to use to whiten as well as clean. With that in mind, however, you may need to increase the amount of baking soda (even more than the extra added teaspoon) in order to get the paste to the consistency you want it to be.

Always stir your paste before use, and check on the consistency. You can add more of any one ingredient at any time, even if you have already used some.

Easy Breezy Whitening Wonder

What you will need:

10 drops myrrh

10 drops spearmint oil

5 drops tea tree oil

1 extra teaspoon baking soda

1 teaspoon hydrogen peroxide

Toothpaste base

Directions:

Combine all of the ingredients in a bowl, mixing well. Make sure your toothpaste base has been thoroughly mixed before you add in the oils, as there are times when the base remains lumpy, and that is difficult to use to brush with. Once combined, transfer into a small, watertight jar until you are ready to use!

To use, simply dip your toothbrush in the paste and brush as you normally would, then rinse and spit when you are done.

Winter Blast

What you will need:

10 drops peppermint oil

10 drops spearmint oil

5 drops cinnamon oil

1 extra teaspoon baking soda

1 teaspoon hydrogen peroxide

Toothpaste base

Directions:

Combine all of the ingredients in a bowl, mixing well. Make sure your toothpaste base has been thoroughly mixed before you add in the oils, as there are times when the base remains lumpy, and that is difficult to use to brush with. Once combined, transfer into a small, watertight jar until you are ready to use!

To use, simply dip your toothbrush in the paste and brush as you normally would, then rinse and spit when you are done.

The White Out

What you will need:

10 drops cinnamon oil

5 drops myrrh oil

5 drops ginger oil

1 teaspoon hydrogen peroxide

Toothpaste base

Toothpaste base

Directions:

Combine all of the ingredients in a bowl, mixing well. Make sure your toothpaste base has been thoroughly mixed before you add in the oils, as there are times when the base remains lumpy, and that is difficult to use to brush with. Once combined, transfer into a small, watertight jar until you are ready to use!

To use, simply dip your toothbrush in the paste and brush as you normally would, then rinse and spit when you are done.

The Dine and Shine

What you will need:

10 drops lemongrass oil

10 drops tea tree oil

5 drops spearmint oil

1 extra teaspoon baking soda

1 teaspoon hydrogen peroxide

Toothpaste base

Directions:

Combine all of the ingredients in a bowl, mixing well. Make sure your toothpaste base has been thoroughly mixed before you add in the oils, as there are times when the base remains lumpy, and that is difficult to use to brush with. Once combined, transfer into a small, watertight jar until you are ready to use!

To use, simply dip your toothbrush in the paste and brush as you normally would, then rinse and spit when you are done.

The Lighthouse

What you will need:

10 drops orange oil

10 drops lemon oil

5 drops clove oil

1 extra teaspoon of baking soda

1 teaspoon hydrogen peroxide

Toothpaste base

Directions:

Combine all of the ingredients in a bowl, mixing well. Make sure your toothpaste base has been thoroughly mixed before you add in the oils, as there are times when the base remains lumpy, and that is difficult to use to brush with. Once combined, transfer into a small, watertight jar until you are ready to use!

To use, simply dip your toothbrush in the paste and brush as you normally would, then rinse and spit when you are done.

Starry Eyes

What you will need:

10 drops lemon oil

10 drops myrrh oil

5 drops spearmint oil

1 extra teaspoon baking soda

1 teaspoon hydrogen peroxide

Toothpaste base

Directions:

Combine all of the ingredients in a bowl, mixing well. Make sure your toothpaste base has been thoroughly mixed before you add in the oils, as there are times when the base remains lumpy, and that is difficult to use to brush with. Once combined, transfer into a small, watertight jar until you are ready to use!

To use, simply dip your toothbrush in the paste and brush as you normally would, then rinse and spit when you are done.

Chapter 3 – For the Kids

There are definitely times when it feels like pulling teeth to get your kids to brush theirs. With these pastes, you won't have an issue getting any one of your kids to do their teeth after lunch, after dinner, or even first thing in the morning.

Whip up any one of these pastes right now, and enjoy the stress less night you are going to have with your kids happy to not only brush their teeth, but also their tongues and gums as well.

Wonderkids

What you will need:

10 drops grapefruit oil

10 drops lemon oil

5 drops peppermint oil

Toothpaste base

Directions:

Combine all of the ingredients in a bowl, mixing well. Make sure your toothpaste base has been thoroughly mixed before you add in the oils, as there are times when the base remains lumpy, and that is difficult to use to brush with. Once combined, transfer into a small, watertight jar until you are ready to use!

To use, simply dip your toothbrush in the paste and brush as you normally would, then rinse and spit when you are done.

The Super Hero Smile

What you will need:

10 drops grapefruit oil

5 drops peppermint oil

5 drops spearmint oil

Toothpaste base

Directions:

Combine all of the ingredients in a bowl, mixing well. Make sure your toothpaste base has been thoroughly mixed before you add in the oils, as there are times when the base remains lumpy, and that is difficult to use to brush with. Once combined, transfer into a small, watertight jar until you are ready to use!

To use, simply dip your toothbrush in the paste and brush as you normally would, then rinse and spit when you are done.

The Twice a Day

What you will need:

10 drops cinnamon oil

5 drops ginger oil

5 drops tea tree oil

Toothpaste base

Directions:

Combine all of the ingredients in a bowl, mixing well. Make sure your toothpaste base has been thoroughly mixed before you add in the oils, as there are times when the base remains lumpy, and that is difficult to use to brush with. Once combined, transfer into a small, watertight jar until you are ready to use!

To use, simply dip your toothbrush in the paste and brush as you normally would, then rinse and spit when you are done.

The ABCs of 123s

What you will need:

10 drops cinnamon oil

10 drops orange oil

1 teaspoon extra baking soda

Toothpaste base

Directions:

Combine all of the ingredients in a bowl, mixing well. Make sure your toothpaste base has been thoroughly mixed before you add in the oils, as there are times when the base remains lumpy, and that is difficult to use to brush with. Once combined, transfer into a small, watertight jar until you are ready to use!

To use, simply dip your toothbrush in the paste and brush as you normally would, then rinse and spit when you are done.

Giggles and Smiles

What you will need:

5 drops grapefruit oil

5 drops lemon oil

5 drops orange oil

5 drops tea tree oil

Toothpaste base

Directions:

Combine all of the ingredients in a bowl, mixing well. Make sure your toothpaste base has been thoroughly mixed before you add in the oils, as there are times when the base remains lumpy, and that is difficult to use to brush with. Once combined, transfer into a small, watertight jar until you are ready to use!

To use, simply dip your toothbrush in the paste and brush as you normally would, then rinse and spit when you are done.

Bright Whites

What you will need:

10 drops peppermint oil

10 drops spearmint oil

5 drops cinnamon oil

1 teaspoon extra baking soda

1 teaspoon hydrogen peroxide

Toothpaste base

Directions:

Combine all of the ingredients in a bowl, mixing well. Make sure your toothpaste base has been thoroughly mixed before you add in the oils, as there are times when the base remains lumpy, and that is difficult to use to brush with. Once combined, transfer into a small, watertight jar until you are ready to use!

To use, simply dip your toothbrush in the paste and brush as you normally would, then rinse and spit when you are done.

Insider's tip:

The hydrogen peroxide may change the consistency of the paste, so you may need to add in a few extra items such as more baking soda, or some extra coconut oil. Play around with it and see what you can come up with.

Chapter 4 – Healthy Gums

They say there is so much more to a smile than just the teeth. You want to have healthy gums and your tongue is no stranger, either. With these pastes, your gums are the star of the show, along with those pearly whites, of course.

The All In One

What you will need:

10 drops tea tree oil

10 drops clove oil

10 drops myrrh oil

Toothpaste base

Directions:

Combine all of the ingredients in a bowl, mixing well. Make sure your toothpaste base has been thoroughly mixed before you add in the oils, as there are times when the base remains lumpy, and that is difficult to use to brush with. Once combined, transfer into a small, watertight jar until you are ready to use!

To use, simply dip your toothbrush in the paste and brush as you normally would, then rinse and spit when you are done.

Pinkys

What you will need:

10 drop grapefruit oil

5 drops tea tree oil

5 drops lemon oil

Toothpaste base

Directions:

Combine all of the ingredients in a bowl, mixing well. Make sure your toothpaste base has been thoroughly mixed before you add in the oils, as there are times when the base remains lumpy, and that is difficult to use to brush with. Once combined, transfer into a small, watertight jar until you are ready to use!

To use, simply dip your toothbrush in the paste and brush as you normally would, then rinse and spit when you are done.

The Perfectionist

What you will need:

10 drops lavender oil

5 drops lemon oil

5 drops wild orange oil

5 drops frankincense oil

Toothpaste base

Directions:

Combine all of the ingredients in a bowl, mixing well. Make sure your toothpaste base has been thoroughly mixed before you add in the oils, as there are times when the base remains lumpy, and that is difficult to use to brush with. Once combined, transfer into a small, watertight jar until you are ready to use!

To use, simply dip your toothbrush in the paste and brush as you normally would, then rinse and spit when you are done.

The Mad Rad

What you will need:

10 drops orange oil

10 drops lemongrass oil

10 drops lemon oil

5 drops clove oil

Toothpaste base

Directions:

Combine all of the ingredients in a bowl, mixing well. Make sure your toothpaste base has been thoroughly mixed before you add in the oils, as there are times when the base remains lumpy, and that is difficult to use to brush with. Once combined, transfer into a small, watertight jar until you are ready to use!

To use, simply dip your toothbrush in the paste and brush as you normally would, then rinse and spit when you are done.

The Complete Package

What you will need:

10 drops peppermint oil

10 drops tea tree oil

10 drops grapefruit oil

10 drops cinnamon oil

10 drops clove oil

1 tablespoon extra baking soda, adjusted to your own taste

Toothpaste base

Directions:

Combine all of the ingredients in a bowl, mixing well. Make sure your toothpaste base has been thoroughly mixed before you add in the oils, as there are times when the base remains lumpy, and that is difficult to use to brush with. Once combined, transfer into a small, watertight jar until you are ready to use!

To use, simply dip your toothbrush in the paste and brush as you normally would, then rinse and spit when you are done.

Heart and Soul

What you will need:

10 drops cinnamon oil

10 drops clove oil

5 drops frankincense oil

5 drops myrrh oil

Extra baking soda to make the proper texture suited to your own particular taste

Toothpaste base

Directions:

Combine all of the ingredients in a bowl, mixing well. Make sure your toothpaste base has been thoroughly mixed before you add in the oils, as there are times when the base remains lumpy, and that is difficult to use to brush with. Once combined, transfer into a small, watertight jar until you are ready to use!

To use, simply dip your toothbrush in the paste and brush as you normally would, then rinse and spit when you are done.

Chapter 5 – Anytime Toothpastes

Whether you want to mix up your routine, or if you are looking for that extra bit of spice to save your night, these are the toothpastes for you. Use them for a date, because you want to change it up, or just because!

The Mix Up

What you will need:

10 drops spearmint oil

10 drops lavender oil

5 drops rose oil

5 drops lemongrass oil

Toothpaste base

Directions:

Combine all of the ingredients in a bowl, mixing well. Make sure your toothpaste base has been thoroughly mixed before you add in the oils, as there are times when the base remains lumpy, and that is difficult to use to brush with. Once combined, transfer into a small, watertight jar until you are ready to use!

To use, simply dip your toothbrush in the paste and brush as you normally would, then rinse and spit when you are done.

One For The Money

What you will need:

10 drops goldenseal oil

5 drops cinnamon oil

5 drops clove oil

Toothpaste base

Directions:

Combine all of the ingredients in a bowl, mixing well. Make sure your toothpaste base has been thoroughly mixed before you add in the oils, as there are times when the base remains lumpy, and that is difficult to use to brush with. Once combined, transfer into a small, watertight jar until you are ready to use!

To use, simply dip your toothbrush in the paste and brush as you normally would, then rinse and spit when you are done.

Wine and Dine

What you will need:

10 drops lavender oil

10 drops spearmint oil

5 drops lemon oil

Toothpaste base

Directions:

Combine all of the ingredients in a bowl, mixing well. Make sure your toothpaste base has been thoroughly mixed before you add in the oils, as there are times when the base remains lumpy, and that is difficult to use to brush with. Once combined, transfer into a small, watertight jar until you are ready to use!

To use, simply dip your toothbrush in the paste and brush as you normally would, then rinse and spit when you are done.

Kiss Me

What you will need:

10 drops cinnamon oil

10 drops rose oil

10 drops clove oil

5 drops tea tree oil

Extra baking soda to your preference

Toothpaste base

Directions:

Combine all of the ingredients in a bowl, mixing well. Make sure your toothpaste base has been thoroughly mixed before you add in the oils, as there are times when the base remains lumpy, and that is difficult to use to brush with. Once combined, transfer into a small, watertight jar until you are ready to use!

To use, simply dip your toothbrush in the paste and brush as you normally would, then rinse and spit when you are done.

The Date Night

What you will need:

10 drops tea tree oil

10 drops eucalyptus oil

5 drops orange oil

Toothpaste base

Directions:

Combine all of the ingredients in a bowl, mixing well. Make sure your toothpaste base has been thoroughly mixed before you add in the oils, as there are times when the base remains lumpy, and that is difficult to use to brush with. Once combined, transfer into a small, watertight jar until you are ready to use!

To use, simply dip your toothbrush in the paste and brush as you normally would, then rinse and spit when you are done.

The Flash

What you will need:

10 drops ginger oil

10 drops eucalyptus

10 drops cinnamon oil

Extra baking soda to your own taste

Toothpaste base

Directions:

Combine all of the ingredients in a bowl, mixing well. Make sure your toothpaste base has been thoroughly mixed before you add in the oils, as there are times when the base remains lumpy, and that is difficult to use to brush with. Once combined, transfer into a small, watertight jar until you are ready to use!

To use, simply dip your toothbrush in the paste and brush as you normally would, then rinse and spit when you are done.

Conclusion

There you have it, everything you need to make your own toothpaste, no matter what kind of teeth you have, or what kind of teeth you want. You may have seen that you should have whiter teeth, even the whitest teeth of all could stand to be a little whiter, or perhaps you are self conscious about your breath... this is the toothpaste for you!

You can make toothpaste that is custom to the need that you have, or you can mix and match the oils with the benefits that you want to make the best toothpaste of all. Of course, I suggest that you make a few different kinds and use them at different times. There's no need to spend all of your efforts on the one kind of toothpaste when you have a variety of different things in your mouth.

This is the book that promotes complete health, no matter what you are looking at. Whiter, brighter, and always better, this is the book that is going to point you in the right direction for the smile of a lifetime. Look no further for your perfect paste.

This is the book that listens to what you need, and gives you that very thing. No mess, no stress, and no hassle. I know you want to have it all, and when you are using the toothpastes in this book, you are going to get that very thing. This is the book for you for any of your oral needs.

I hope you see the other benefits that come from using this toothpaste as well. I know that you are using it in your mouth, but it won't be long before you gain the other health benefits that come with the use of these oils, including better health itself!

So many essential oils have a variety of health benefits, and it's hard to get one without all the others. This is your chance to make a major impact on your health with only a miner change in your day. I hope you get all of what you are looking for and more with this book, and that all of your oral needs are met without any more searching or trying.

You're smile is worth a million dollars, and now you can get out there and smile like you mean it.